Menopause Diet

22 Mouth Watering Recipes for Menopause

Table of Contents

Introduction

Menopause is a normal part of aging for women and no women can escape it. There are certain symptoms that are associated with menopause, including night sweats, hot flashes, mood swings, depression, joint pain, low sex drive, and weight gain.

Recent medical research has revealed that many of the unpleasant symptoms that women associate with the menopause are the result of a standard Western diet. Data shows that one in every two women entering menopause is overweight and at risk for diabetes, high blood pressure, heart disease and stroke. However, if you take certain steps, including some lifestyle changes and change the way you eat, you can effectively manage your weight gain during your menopause.

With an appropriate diet plan, it is also possible for women to lose weight during and after menopause. Following a healthy diet that includes mainly low-calorie, nutrient-rich foods can help you balance your intake for weight control and help you meet your nutrient needs at the same time. The book offers easy to make, mouthwatering recipes that will help you get through these difficult times with relative ease.

Chapter 1 Healthy Eating During Menopause

It is important to eat a healthy, balanced diet during your menopause. You should eat a wide variety of foods in the right proportions. The following is a basic guideline for menopause diet.

- Get enough fiber: Eat foods that are high in fiber, such as rice, pasta, cereals, whole-grain bread, vegetables, and fresh fruits. Most adult women should get about 21 gram of fiber daily.

- Pump up your iron: Eat at least three servings of iron-rich foods daily. Iron is found in fish, poultry, lean red meat, eggs, enriched grain products, nuts and leafy green vegetables. It is recommended that older women take 8 milligrams of iron daily.

- Get enough calcium: Eat and drink two to four servings of calcium-rich foods such as dairy products daily. Calcium is found in fish with bones, broccoli, legumes, and in dairy products. Try to get 1,200 milligrams of calcium daily.

- Focus on fruits and vegetables; Eat at least 2 cups of vegetables and 1 ½ cups of fruit daily.

- Read labels: Read labels whenever buying packaged foods to help yourself make better food choices.

- Avoid high-fat foods: Avoid high-fat foods such as fatty meats, whole milk, ice cream. Avoid trans fats found in vegetable oils, baked goods, and some margarine.

- Use sugar and salt in moderation.

- Limit alcohol to one glass of wine, one beer or 1 ounce of spirits daily.

Other lifestyle changes

- If you smoke, then quit.

- Exercise 30 minutes three to five times a week.

- Vitamin D: Your body needs vitamin D to absorb calcium. People ages 51 to 70 should get 600 IU daily. 15 to 20 minutes of midday sun exposure is an excellent way to get enough quality vitamin D. Don't get scared of over sun exposure because 15 to 20 minutes of daily sun exposure wouldn't cause any skin health problem.

Here is a list of foods to avoid and foods that help in menopause moments

- Memory lapses: Antioxidant-rich foods such as vegetables and blueberries help slow down memory lapses. Also, skipping meals can affect your memory and concentration.

- o Achy joints: Avoid caffeinated drinks and eat omega-3 rich foods such as salmon.

- o Headaches: Avoid MSG and alcohol. Eat magnesium-rich foods such as black beans and almonds.

- o Mood swings: Avoid sugar-rich foods and drinks, such as sweetened soda, candy, and doughnuts. Eat asparagus, beets, Brussels sprouts to relieve depression.

- o Hot flashes: Avoid large meals, hot beverages, and alcohol. Add soy foods to your diet.

A few eating tips

- o Eat mindfully. Eat slowly, chew your food and enjoy your food.

- o Listen to your body. Stop eating when you start to feel full.

- o Know when to eat. Eat large meal between 11 AM and 2 PM.

- o Eat healthy snacks. Eat a healthy snack in the late afternoon (such as a banana or a few nuts) to keep your energy up and prevent overeating at dinner.

CHAPTER 2
BREAKFAST
RECIPES

Cranberry Muffins

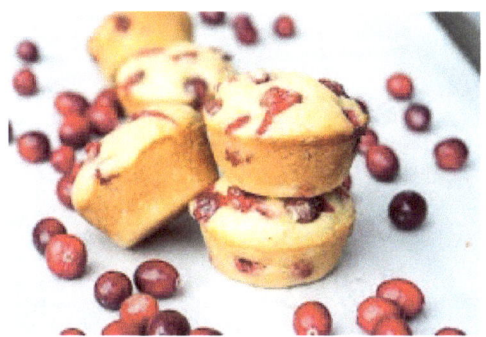

Ingredients for 8 muffins

- o All-purpose flour – ¾ cup
- o Sugar – 1/3 cup
- o Baking powder – 2 teaspoons
- o Baking soda – ½ teaspoon
- o Pinch of salt
- o Ground cinnamon – ¾ teaspoon
- o Unprocessed miller's wheat bran – 1 cup
- o 1% milk – ½ cup
- o Egg – 1
- o Oil – 2 tablespoons
- o Chopped fresh cranberries – ½ cup

Method

1. Preheat the oven to 400F and line eight standard muffin cups with paper baking

cups. If desired, sprinkle very lightly with raw sugar.

2. In a medium-size mixing bowl, combine the sugar, baking powder, flour, baking soda, cinnamon, wheat bran and salt and mix well. In another bowl, combine the egg, oil, milk and cranberries and mix well. Make a well in the center of the dry ingredients and pour in the wet ingredients. Mix until just combine.

3. Fill the muffin cups about ¾ full with the batter and bake until a toothpick inserted in the center comes out clean, about 10 to 20 minutes.

Nutrition Facts Per Serving

- Cal 100
- GI 65
- Carb 16 g
- Fiber 4 g
- Protein 3 g
- Sodium 281 mg

GI – Glycemic Index

Mushroom and Egg Breakfast

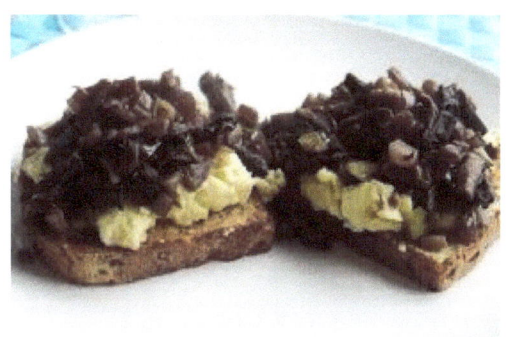

Ingredients for 2 servings

- o   Whole-grain bread – 2 slices

- o   Olive oil margarine – 1 teaspoon

- o   Button mushrooms – 1 ½ ounces (about 4), stems trimmed, sliced

- o   Large spinach leaves – 3 large, washed and chopped

- o   Freshly ground pepper

- o   Egg – 2

- o   Coarsely grated reduced-fat Cheddar cheese - 1 tablespoon

- o   Olive oil cooking spray

Method

1.   Preheat the oven to 350F.

2.   Cut the crusts off the bread and spray both sides of each slice lightly with oil. Into two 1/3 cup capacity nonstick

muffin cups, press the bread slices firmly. Set aside.

3. In a nonstick skillet, heat the margarine over medium-high heat until sizzling. Add the mushrooms and cook until tender, about 4 to 5 minutes, stir often. Now add the spinach and cook, until wilted, about 1 to 2 minutes, stirring often. Remove from the heat and season with pepper to taste.

4. Over each of the muffin cups of bread, spoon half the mushroom mixture and press lightly. In a small dish, crack an egg and then slide it on top of the mushrooms. Repeat the remaining egg and muffin cup, then sprinkle with cheese.

5. Bake until the egg is cooked to your liking. 15 minutes for a softly set yolk and 20 minutes for a hard-cooked yolk.

6. Serve.

Nutrition Facts Per Serving

- Cal 175
- GI 67
- Carb 13 g
- Fiber 2.5 g
- Protein 12 g
- Sodium 257 mg

Egg Scramble

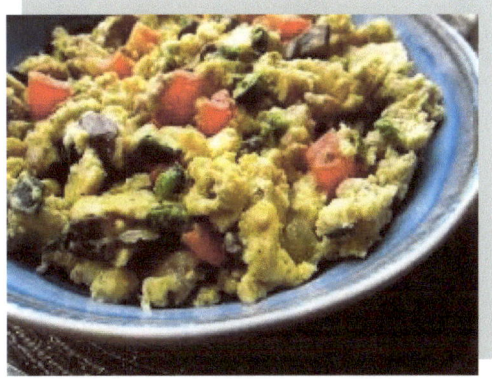

Ingredients for 1 serving

- o   Small fingerling potatoes – 5 or 6
- o   Extra-virgin olive oil – 1 teaspoon
- o   Diced white onion – 1 to 2 tablespoons
- o   Garlic clove – 1, minced
- o   Canned black beans – ¼ to 1/3 cups, drained and rinsed
- o   Eggs – 2
- o   Ground cumin – ½ teaspoon
- o   Salt and pepper
- o   Tabasco sauce – 2 to 20 dashes
- o   Diced avocado and tomato (optional)

Method

1.   In a microwave-safe bowl, place a few drops of water. Prick your potatoes with

a fork before cooking if your potatoes are thick.

2. Place the potatoes in the bowl, cover with plastic wrap and cook on high until the potatoes are tender, about 3 to 4 minutes. Alternatively, you can peel the potatoes and boil in water until tender. Slice them in half and set aside.

3. Heat the olive oil over medium heat in a stainless-steel saucepan. Add the onion and sauté for 3 minutes, then add the potatoes and sauté for 1 minute more. Add the garlic and sauté for another minute. Now add the beans and sauté for 2 minutes more.

4. Into a small bowl, break the eggs. Season with cumin, salt, and pepper, then beat with a fork. Add to the bean mixture and cook for 1 minute or more to your desired consistency.

5. Add Tabasco sauce and top with diced avocado and tomato.

Nutrition Facts Per Serving

- o   Cal 503

- o   GI 66

- o   Carb 58 g

- o   Fiber 2 g

- o   Protein 22 g

- o   Sodium 419 mg

Whole-Grain Pancakes

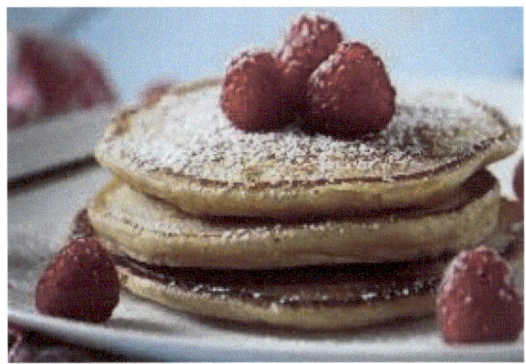

Ingredients for 4 servings

- o   Whole wheat flour – ½ cup
- o   Sifted all-purpose flour – ¼ cup
- o   Soy protein powder – 3 tablespoons
- o   Non-aluminum baking powder – 2 teaspoons
- o   Salt – ¼ teaspoon
- o   Soy milk or water - 1 1/3 cups
- o   Oil – 2 tablespoons
- o   Cooking spray

Method

1. In a medium-size bowl, mix together the soy protein powder, flours, baking powder, and salt. Add the oil and soy milk and stir just until blended.

2. Spray a large skillet with cooking spray and heat over medium-high heat. Onto the hot pan, spoon the batter, ¼ cup for each pancake. Cook about 2 minutes, or until evenly covered with bubbles. Then carefully turn over with a spatula and cook for another 2 minutes, or until lightly browned. Repeat with the remaining batter.

Nutrition Facts Per Serving

- Cal 237

- GI 62

- Carb 32 g

- Fiber 3 g

- Protein 9 g

- Sodium 488 mg

Wild Blueberry Granola French Toast

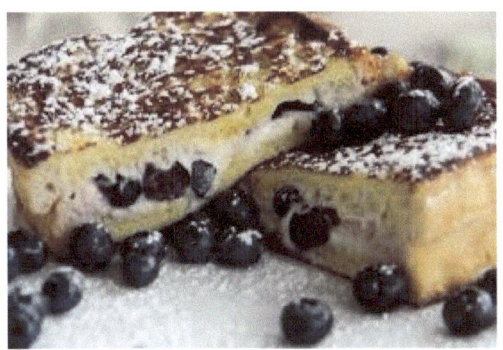

Ingredients for 2 servings

Batter

- o   Milk – ¼ cup
- o   Sugar – 2 tablespoons
- o   Eggs – 2, separated

French Toast

- o   Butter – 2 tablespoons
- o   Wild Maine blueberry granola – 1 cup, ground coarsely
- o   Brioche toast – 2 (1-inch-thick) slices

Method

1.   Preheat the oven to 450F.

2. Make the batter – in a bowl, whip the egg whites until they form a soft peak. Add the sugar at the end. Whisk the yolks and the milk together in a separate bowl. Into the yolk mixture, gently fold 1/3 of the whites. Then fold the remaining whites into the mixture in two separate stages.

3. Make the French toast – dip the toast slices into the batter so they are coated evenly. Sprinkle the tops evenly with the granola.

4. In an ovenproof skillet, heat the butter over medium-high heat. Place the slices of toast in the skillet until golden brown on the bottom, about 4 to 5 minutes. Then flip the toast slices over and place the pan in the oven for 3 to 4 minutes to finish cooking.

5. Serve.

Nutrition Facts Per Serving

- Cal 468
- GI 62
- Carb 67 g
- Fiber 5 g
- Protein 15 g
- Sodium 334 mg

CHAPTER 3
SOUPS

Crab and Sweet Potato Soup

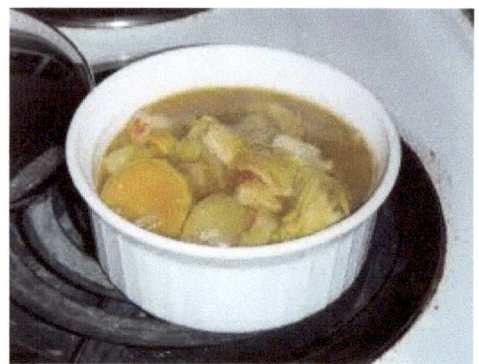

Ingredients for 6 to 8 servings

- o   Sweet potatoes – 2 pounds, peeled and diced
- o   Yellow onion – 1/2, diced
- o   Garlic – 4 cloves, minced
- o   Ground coriander – 1 tablespoon
- o   Salt – 1 teaspoon
- o   Grated nutmeg – 1 teaspoon
- o   Cayenne – ½ teaspoon
- o   Ground white pepper – ½ teaspoon
- o   Cloves – 2, whole
- o   Dry sherry – 1 ½ cups
- o   Orange juice – 1 cup
- o   Lemon juice – ¼ cup
- o   Hoisin sauce – 1 tablespoon
- o   Crabmeat – 1 pound (claw)

Method

1. Except for the crab, combine all the ingredients in a large saucepan with 8 cups of water. Cover and bring just to a boil over medium-high heat, and then lower the heat and simmer, covered, until the potatoes are tender, about 20 to 30 minutes.

2. Puree the soup with an immersion blender. Add the crabmeat and heat through.

3. Serve.

Nutrition Facts Per Serving

- Cal 235

- GI 50

- Carb 30.5 g

- Fiber 3.3 g

- Protein 14 g

- Sodium 382 mg

Apple and Sweet Potato Soup

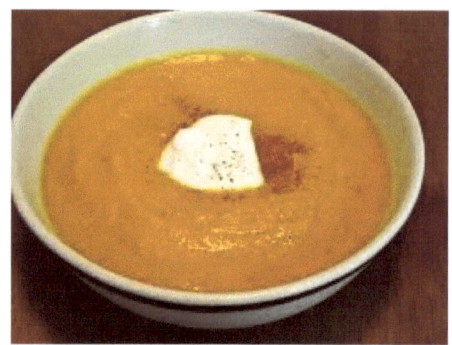

Ingredients for 6 servings

- Medium-size sweet potatoes – 2, peeled and cut into medium-size chunks

- Firm apple – 1 (Jonagold or Gala), peeled, cored and quartered

- Yellow onion – 1, medium, peeled and quartered

- Garlic – 2 cloves

- Olive oil – 2 tablespoons

- Salt and pepper

- Low-sodium chicken or vegetable broth – 3 to 4 cups

- Nonfat sour cream – ¾ cup, for serving

Method

1. Preheat the oven to 450F.

2. In a roasting pan, put the sweet potatoes, onion, apples and garlic.

Drizzle with olive oil and sprinkle with salt and pepper to taste.

3. Place in the oven and roast, for 30 minutes, or until the apples and vegetables are tender, toss every 10 minutes.

4. Add just enough broth to cover the mixture and puree using an immersion blender. Add more broth if necessary.

5. In a saucepan, warm the soup over low heat until ready to serve.

6. If desired, stir in the sour cream for a creamier taste.

Nutrition Facts Per Serving

- Cal 145
- GI 54
- Carb 23 g
- Fiber 2 g
- Protein 4 g
- Sodium 427 mg

Italian-Style Vegetable and Bean Soup

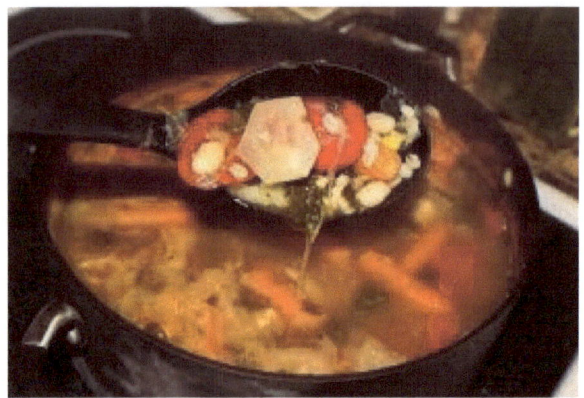

Ingredients for 6 main-dish or 12 side-dish

- o   Extra-virgin olive oil – 3 tablespoons

- o   White onion – 1 large, chopped

- o   All-purpose flour – ¼ cup

- o   Dry sherry or dry red wine – 1 cup

- o   Potatoes – 2 large, peeled and cut into ½ -inch cubes

- o   White cabbage – 1 small head, cored and chopped into bite-size pieces

- o   Celery – 2 ribs, chopped

- o   Zucchini – 2, cut into ½ - inch cubes

- o   Tomatoes – 2 large, chopped

- o   Cooked white beans – 1 cup

- o   Cooked chickpeas – 1 cup

- o   Low-sodium chicken or vegetable broth

- ○ Salt and pepper

- ○ Fresh basil – 1 teaspoon, chopped

- ○ Bay leaf – 1

- ○ Fresh Italian parsley – ½ bunch, chopped

- ○ Raw rice – 1 cup or ½ pound pasta shells (optional)

Method

1. In a large saucepan, heat the olive oil over medium heat. Add the onion and sauté until translucent, but not browned. Whisk in the flour to make a roux.

2. To the saucepan, add beans (drain and rinse the beans, if using canned), tomatoes, zucchini, celery, cabbage, potatoes, and sherry. Add enough broth to cover and bring to a boil. Skim off any froth that rises to the surface.

3. Skim off all the froth, then lower the heat to low and season with salt and pepper.

4. Add the parsley, bay leaf and basil and simmer, covered, until the vegetables are tender, but not mushy.

5. When the vegetables are done add the rice or pasta if desired, and cook until al dente.

6. Pour on individual bowls. Drizzle with extra-virgin olive oil and serve.

Nutrition Facts Per Serving

- ○ Cal 525
- ○ GI 54
- ○ Carb 87 g
- ○ Fiber 11 g
- ○ Protein 16 g
- ○ Sodium 670 mg

CHAPTER 4
MAIN
MEALS

Haddock with Tomatoes

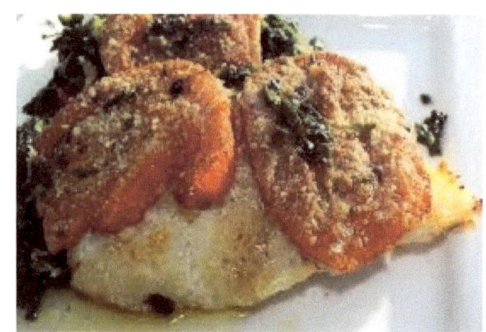

Ingredients for 1 serving

- o Haddock fillet – 1 (1/2 – pound)
- o Olive oil -2 teaspoons
- o Freshly ground pepper – 1/8 teaspoon
- o Minced shallot – ½ tablespoon
- o Halved cherry tomatoes – ½ cup
- o Chopped olives – 1/8 cup
- o Capers – ½ tablespoon, rinsed and chopped
- o Dried oregano – 1 teaspoon
- o Balsamic vinegar – ½ teaspoon

Method

1. Preheat the oven to 450F.

2. Use 1 teaspoon olive oil to rub the haddock fillet, sprinkle with pepper and place in a small roasting pan.

3. Bake until the fish easily flake with a fork, about 15 minutes.

4. While the fish is roasting, in a skillet, heat the remaining teaspoon of olive oil over medium-high heat. Add the shallot and sauté for 20 seconds. Then add the capers, olives, and tomatoes and sauté for about 30 seconds. Then stir in the vinegar and oregano. Set aside and keep warm.

5. Once the haddock is cooked, place on a plate. Top with warm tapenade and serve.

Nutrition Facts Per Serving

- Cal 263
- GI 51
- Carb 9 g
- Fiber 3 g
- Protein 44 g
- Sodium 463 mg

Citrusy Trout

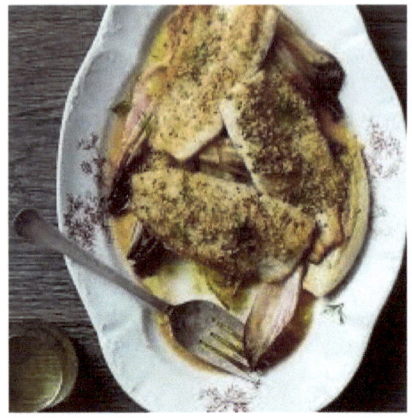

Ingredients for 4 servings

Seasoning

- o   Salt – 1 ½ tablespoons

- o   Chili powder – 1 teaspoon

- o   Ground cumin – ½ teaspoon

- o   Ground coriander – ½ teaspoon

Fish

- o   Cooking spray

- o   Sunburst trout fillets – 4 (6-ounce)

- o   Ruby red grapefruit section – 1, quartered

- o   Navel orange sections – 2, halved

- o   Blood orange sections – 2, halved

- o   Satsuma sections – 4

- o   Orange marmalade – ½ cup

- Green onions – 2, sliced diagonally
- Fresh cilantro – 4 sprigs

Method

1. To make the seasoning, combine the coriander, chili powder, cumin and salt and store in a spice bottle.

2. Preheat the oven to 400F. Spray a baking dish with cooking spray.

3. Season each fish fillet with ¼ teaspoon of the seasoning. Bake or grill the fish until cooked through, about 10 to 12 minutes.

4. Meanwhile, divide the citrus sections equally among four small bowls and add 2 tablespoons of the marinade to each bowl.

5. To serve, place a fillet of fish on individual serving plates. Top each with green onions, citrus sections mixture and a sprig of cilantro.

Nutrition Facts Per Serving

- Cal 489
- GI 44
- Carb 60 g
- Fiber 6 g
- Protein 38 g
- Sodium 2980 mg

Halibut with Black Chickpea

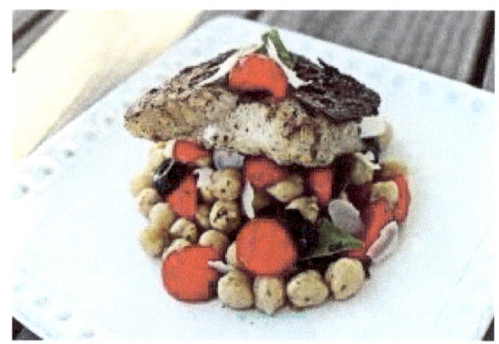

Ingredients for 6 servings

- o Black chickpeas – 2 ½ cups (soaked overnight)
- o Low-sodium chicken or vegetable broth – 4 quarts
- o Onion -1, halved
- o Carrot – 1
- o Garlic – 1 clove
- o Pork (bacon, ham hock, prosciutto) – 1 piece (2-ounce)
- o Olive oil – 3 tablespoons
- o Ripe tomatoes – 2, diced
- o Red bell pepper -1, roasted, seeded, peeled and diced
- o Black olives – 12, chopped
- o Zest of 2 lemons
- o White balsamic vinegar - 6 tablespoons
- o Shallots – 4, chopped

- Fresh parsley -1 bunch, chopped
- Salt and pepper
- Olive oil – 4 quarts
- Halibut – 6 thick pieces (6-ounce)

Method

1. In a large, heavy saucepan, place the chickpeas. Add the onion, carrot, garlic, broth, and pork. Bring to a boil and then lower the heat and simmer, covered, until the beans are tender, about 1 to 2 hours. Drain and put the chickpeas in a large bowl. Discard the carrot, garlic, onion, and pork.

2. In a large saucepan, heat the olive oil over medium-high heat. Add the roasted bell pepper, olives, tomatoes, vinegar, shallots, lemon zest, and parsley and sauté until the vegetables are tender. Add the mixture to the bowl of chickpeas. Season with salt and pepper to taste. Set aside in a warm place.

Nutrition Facts Per Serving

- Cal 6040
- GI 45
- Carb 60 g
- Fiber 15 g
- Protein 67 g
- Sodium 2863 mg

Sweet and Sour Tuna

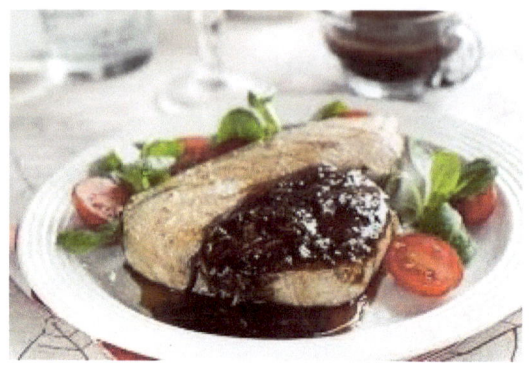

Ingredients for 4 servings

- o   Tuna steaks – 4
- o   All-purpose flour for coating
- o   Salt
- o   Extra- virgin olive oil – 3 tablespoons
- o   Large onion – 1, sliced
- o   Red wine vinegar – ½ cup
- o   Marsala – 3 tablespoons
- o   Golden raisins – ½ cup
- o   Pitted green olives – 12 large
- o   Bay leaves – 3

Method

1. Rinse the tuna steaks. Pat dry and then coat them with the flour and salt.

2. In a large skillet, heat the olive oil over medium heat. Add the onion and sauté

until tender, but not browned. Now add the tuna steaks and cook 4 minutes on each side. Add the Marsala, raisins, vinegar, bay leaves and olives and cook for about 7 minutes.

3. Now turn off the heat, cover the skillet and let rest for 10 minutes, so the flavor of the sauce can be absorbed by the fish. Discard the bay leaves before serving.

Nutrition Facts Per Serving

- o Cal 282
- o GI 63
- o Carb 20 g
- o Fiber 2 g
- o Protein 18 g
- o Sodium 556 mg

Grilled Salmon Skewers

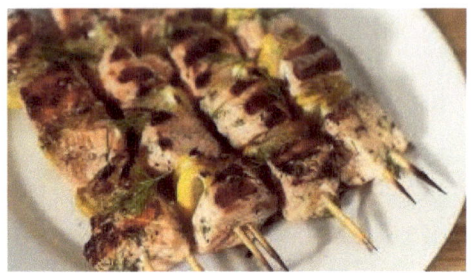

Ingredients for 4 servings

- ○ Salmon fillet – 1 (1-pound), sliced lengthwise into 4 (1-inch) strips

- ○ Soy sauce – ½ cup

- ○ Freshly squeezed orange juice – ½ cup

- ○ Freshly squeezed lime juice – ¼ cup

- ○ Minced ginger – 1 tablespoon

- ○ Garlic clove -1, minced

- ○ Red pepper flakes – 1 teaspoon

- ○ Furikake -1 teaspoon

Method

1. Thread each salmon strip onto a soaked skewer and place in a shallow dish. (Soak four bamboo skewers in water for 30 minutes.)

2. In a bowl, whisk together the furikake, red pepper flakes, garlic, ginger, lime juice, orange juice, and soy sauce. Pour

about ½ cup of the soy juice mixture over the skewers and turn to coat. Marinate for at least 30 minutes. Reserve the remaining marinade for dipping.

3. Preheat an outdoor grill to medium-high heat and oil the grill generously. Cook the skewers until the fish starts to flake, about 2 minutes per side. Brushing often with the marinade. Let them rest for 2 minutes before serving.

4. Serve with reserved marinade on the side.

Nutrition Facts Per Serving

- Cal 200
- GI 45
- Carb 8 g
- Fiber 1 g
- Protein 27 g
- Sodium 1866 mg

Nettles and Scallops with Capers-Raisins Sauce

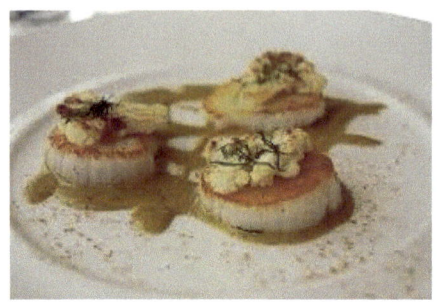

Ingredients for 4 servings

- o Nettles -4, stems removed (wear gloves)
- o Olive oil – 4 tablespoons, divided
- o Water – ¼ cup plus ½ cup
- o Kosher salt as needed
- o Sunchokes -2, peeled and sliced
- o Golden raisins – 2/3 cup
- o Capers – 2 tablespoons
- o Sherry wine vinegar – 2 tablespoons
- o Dry-packed day-boat scallops – 4 large (size U-10)
- o Canola oil – 1 tablespoon
- o Butter – 2 tablespoons

Method

1. Prepare the nettles, in a saucepan, combine 2 tablespoons olive oil, water,

nettles, and salt and cook over medium-low heat until the nettles are tender, about 10 minutes. Set aside.

2. To prepare the sunchokes, in a skillet, heat the olive oil over medium-high heat. Add the sun chokes and sauté until golden brown. Season with salt to taste and set aside.

3. To make the sauce, in a saucepan, put the capers, raisins, vinegar and water and simmer until raisins are rehydrated. Add some water if the mixture becomes too dry. Blend in a food processor and set aside.

4. To make the scallops, season them with salt. In a skillet, heat the canola oil over high heat. Then add the scallops and sauté for 30 seconds. Add the butter and continue to cook until the bottom side of the scallops are golden brown. Then flip the scallops, reduce the heat and cook for another 2 minutes. Remove from the skillet and pat dry.

5. Spoon the sauce onto each of four individual serving plates. Add the nettles and scallops. Top with sun chokes. Serve.

Shrimp with Tomato Sauce

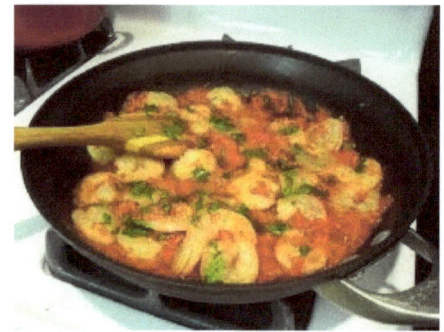

Ingredients for 4 servings

- o   Shrimp – 1 ½ pounds

- o   Extra-virgin olive oil – ½ cup

- o   Medium-size red onion – 1, chopped finely

- o   Garlic – 3 cloves, chopped finely

- o   Celery – 1 large rib, chopped finely

- o   Small carrot – 1, small, pared and chopped finely

- o   Italian tomatoes - 1 (28-ounce) can

- o   Salt and pepper to taste

- o   Raisins – 5 tablespoons

- o   Pine nuts – 5 tablespoons

- o   Capers – 6 tablespoons, drained

- o   Bay leaves – 6

- o   Handful of chopped fresh basil and fresh Italian parsley

- o   Lemon – 1, cut into 4 wedges

Method

1. Preheat the oven to 375F.

2. Wash and drain the shrimp, then set aside in ice-cold water.

3. In a medium-size skillet, heat the olive oil over medium heat. Add the carrot, celery, garlic, and onion and sauté until the vegetables are tender, about 10 minutes. Add the tomatoes, smash them with a wooden spoon and cook for 15 minutes longer. Season with salt and pepper to taste.

4. While the vegetables are cooking, soak the raisins in a small bowl of warm water for 10-12 minutes. Drain. Add the raisins, capers, and pine nuts to the skillet and cook for another 10 minutes.

5. Transfer the tomato-celery mixture to a glass baking dish. Drain the shrimp and place them over the tomato sauce. Now add the bay leaves. Cover the baking dish with aluminum foil and bake for 10 minutes.

6. Remove the dish from the oven, discard the bay leaves and slowly mix the cooked shrimp into the tomato sauce.

7. Serve sprinkled with parsley and basil and with lemon wedges on the side.

Chicken and Shrimp Sorentina

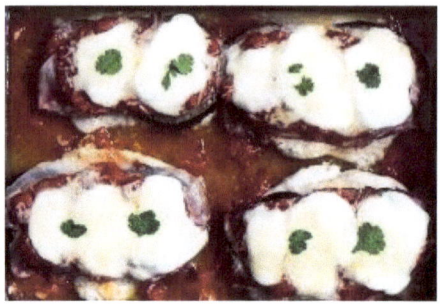

Ingredients for 4 servings

- o   Boneless chicken breasts – 4, pounded thin

- o   All-purpose flour for dredging

- o   Margarine – 1 tablespoon

- o   Jumbo shrimp – 10 to 12

- o   Artichoke hearts – 16 to 20, quartered

- o   Ripe tomato – 1, diced

- o   Rubbed sage – 1 ½ teaspoons

- o   Dried parsley – 1 tablespoon

- o   Dry white wine – 1 cup

- o   Chicken broth – 1 cup

- o   Salt and pepper

- o   Prosciutto – 8 slices

- o   Mozzarella cheese – 8 slices

Method

1. Dredge the chicken in the flour. In a large skillet, heat the margarine over medium heat. Add the shrimp and chicken and sauté until the chicken is browned on one side. Add the tomatoes and artichoke hearts. Turn the chicken breasts and brown on the other side.

2. Add the parsley, sage and wine and simmer for 4 to 5 minutes. Add the broth, lower the heat to low and simmer for a few minutes more. Season with salt and pepper to taste.

3. Top with mozzarella and prosciutto and continue to simmer until the cheese melts. Serve.

Nutrition Facts Per Serving

- o Cal 509
- o GI 49
- o Carb 26 g
- o Fiber 16 g
- o Protein 57 g
- o Sodium 1570 mg

Spicy Chicken over Cranberry-Apricot Couscous

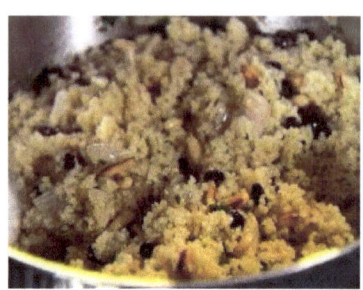

Ingredients for 4 to 6 servings

Chicken

- Ground cinnamon – 1 teaspoon
- Ground cloves – 1 teaspoon
- Cayenne – 1 teaspoon
- Ground cumin – 1 teaspoon
- Fennel seeds – 1 teaspoon
- Sweet paprika – 1 tablespoon
- Kosher salt – ¾ teaspoon
- Brown sugar – 1 teaspoon
- Juice of ½ lemon
- Olive oil – 2 tablespoon
- Garlic cloves – 4, crushed
- Boneless, skinless chicken breasts – 1 ½ to 2 pounds

Couscous

- o   Couscous – 1 cup
- o   Dried apricots – 10
- o   Dried cranberries – ½ cup
- o   Boiling water – 1 ½ cups
- o   Green onions – 2, green parts only, chopped
- o   Fresh cilantro – 2 handfuls, chopped
- o   Juice of ½ lemon
- o   Extra-virgin olive oil – 2 tablespoons
- o   Kosher salt and freshly ground pepper

Method

1. To make the chicken, in a large bowl, combine all ingredients and mix well to make a rich marinade. Add the chicken and marinate for at least 30 minutes.

2. While the chicken marinates, work on the couscous. In a medium-size bowl, add the apricots, cranberries, and couscous and pour the boiling water over them, then stir with a fork to combine. Cover and allow to sit for 10 to 15 minutes. Then uncover and fluff with a fork.

3. Add the cilantro and green onions and drizzle with the olive oil and lemon juice. Season with salt and pepper to taste and toss gently to combine. Set aside and keep warm.

4. To make the dish, heat a grill pan or a skillet over medium heat. Then add the chicken and brown on both sides. Careful not to burn the spice mixture on the chicken.

5. Brown both sides, and turn the heat down to low. Place a lid over the skillet. The lid will allow the chicken to almost steam, which will make a very moist chicken breast.

6. Once the chicken is fully cooked, remove it from the heat and let it rest for 10 minutes. Then slice against the grain. Serve with the couscous.

Nutrition Facts Per Serving (chicken)

- Cal 238
- GI 51
- Carb 4 g
- Fiber 1 g
- Protein 31 g
- Sodium 434 mg

Nutrition Facts Per Serving (couscous)

- Cal 252
- GI 55
- Carb 46 g
- Fiber 4 g
- Protein 6 g

CHAPTER 5
DESSERTS

Stuffed Pears

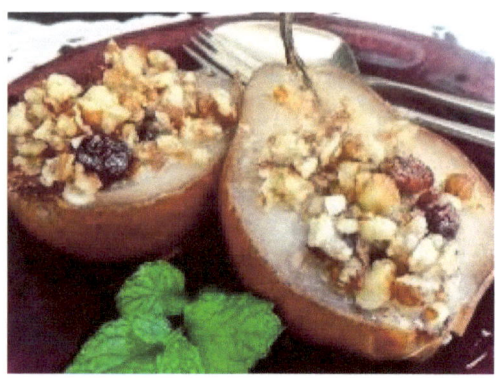

Ingredients for 4 servings

- o   Sliced almonds – ½ cup, toasted and chopped finely

- o   Confectioners' sugar – 1 tablespoon

- o   Ripe pears – 2 large, halved and cored

- o   Dry Marsala wine – 3 tablespoons

Method

1. Preheat the oven to 400F and lightly grease a baking dish with a small amount of butter.

2. Combine the sugar and almonds in a small bowl and mix well.

3. In the greased baking dish, place each pear half so that they fit snugly together. Stuff each pear half with the nut mixture, then pour a little of the Marsala on top of each pear.

4. Bake uncovered for 10 minutes. Serve warm.

Nutrition Facts Per Serving

- Cal 190
- GI 37
- Carb 24 g
- Fiber 5 g
- Protein 4 g
- Sodium 2 mg

Strawberries with Cheese Topping

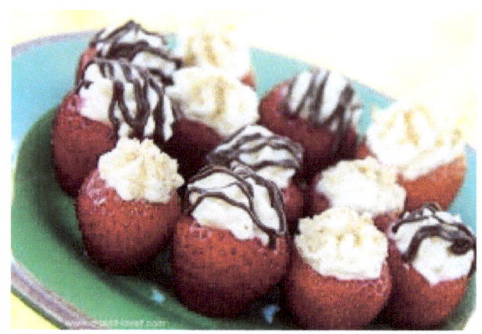

Ingredients for 4 servings

- o Walnuts – ¼ cup, coarsely chopped

- o White chocolate chunks – ¼ cup

- o Nonfat Ricotta cheese – 1 (15-ounce) package, crumbled

- o Light cream cheese – 1 (4-ounce) package

- o Sugar – ¼ cup

- o Vanilla extract – 2 tablespoons

- o Fresh strawberries

Method

1. In a food processor, place the chocolate and walnuts and pulse until the mixture becomes coarse in texture. In a medium-size mixing bowl, place the cheeses, sugar, and vanilla and mix well to combine. Keep in the refrigerator until ready to serve.

2. Cut the strawberries in half and place them in individual serving bowls. On top of the strawberries, place a few spoonsful of the cheese mixture. Sprinkle with the walnut mixture and serve.

Nutrition Facts Per Serving

- Cal 363
- GI 48
- Carb 41 g
- Fiber 4 g
- Protein 21 g
- Sodium 233 mg

Baked Spiced Pears with Sauce

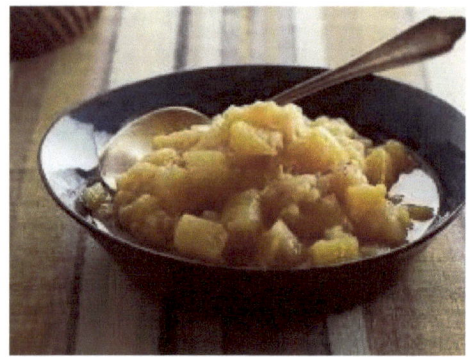

Ingredients for 4 servings

- Ripe Bosc pears – 2, peel, halved and scored
- LoGiCane sugar – 1 tablespoon
- Ground cinnamon – ¼ teaspoon
- Ground cardamom – ¼ teaspoon

Sauce

- Egg yolk – 1
- LoGiCane sugar – 1 tablespoon
- Marsala wine – 2 tablespoons

Method

1. Preheat the oven to 350F.

2. In a rectangular baking dish, place the pears, cut side down with just enough water to cover the bottom of the dish.

3. Combine the spices and sugar and sprinkle half of this mixture over the pears.

4. In the preheated oven, bake the pears for 5 minutes. Turn the pear halves over and sprinkle with the remaining spice mixture. Then bake for another 5 minutes. The pears are done when they are easily pierced with a fork but still, hold their shape. Remove from the oven. Place in individual dessert dishes, and set aside.

5. To make the sauce, in a very small saucepan, combine the sugar and egg yolk. Then with a wooden spoon, mix vigorously for at least 5 minutes. Slowly add the Marsala and mix well.

6. Heat over low heat until the mixture thickens, about 1 minute. Stir constantly. Careful not to boil.

7. Pour the sauce over the pear halves and serve.

Nutrition Facts Per Serving

- o   Cal 99

- o   GI 44

- o   Carb 18 g

- o   Fiber 3 g

- o   Protein 1 g

- o   Sodium 3 mg

Frozen Berry Yogurt

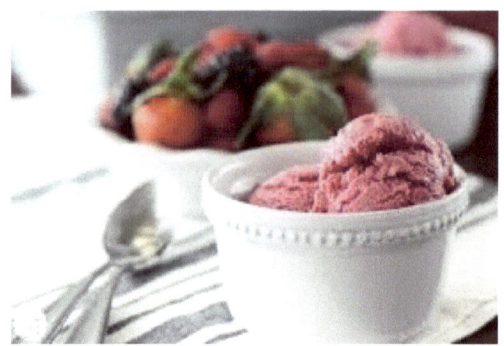

Ingredients for 6 servings

- o Fresh and frozen mixed berries – 9 ounces

- o Low-fat vanilla yogurt – 3 (7-ounce) tubs

- o Egg whites – 2

- o Pure floral honey – 2 tablespoons

Method

1. Place the yogurt and berries in a food processor and blend until smooth. Transfer to a medium-size bowl and set aside.

2. In a clean, dry bowl, whisk the egg whites until stiff peaks form. A tablespoon at a time, add the honey after each addition whisks well until thick and glossy. Fold into the yogurt mixture until just combined.

3. Pour the mixture into an airtight container and place in the freezer until frozen, about 4 hours. Then, with a

metal spoon, break the frozen yogurt into chunks. Blend in the food processor again until smooth. Return to the airtight container and refreeze until frozen, about 3 hours. Serve in scoops.

Nutrition Facts Per Serving

- Cal 126
- GI 43
- Carb 23 g
- Fiber 1 g
- Protein 6 g
- Sodium 85 mg

Chocolate Chip Cookies

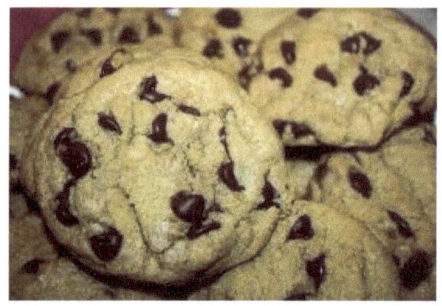

Ingredients for 36 cookies

- o   Rolled oats – 1 cup

- o   Spelt flour – 1 cup

- o   Brown rice flour – ¼ cup

- o   Baking soda – ¼ teaspoon

- o   Fine sea salt – ¼ teaspoon

- o   Safflower oil – ¾ cup

- o   Pure maple syrup – 1 cup

- o   Vanilla extract – ¼ teaspoon

- o   Almond extract – ¼ teaspoon

- o   Egg replacer – 1 tablespoon

- o   Chocolate chips – 1 cup

Method

1. Preheat the oven to 350F.

2. In a large mixing bowl, combine the flours, oats, baking soda and salt. Add ¼ cup of water, oil, almond extracts, vanilla, maple syrup, and egg replacer and stir well to combine.

3. Fold the chocolate chips into the batter. Onto a large baking sheet, spoon tablespoons of batter 3 inches apart. With the back of a wet spoon, flatten the batter.

4. Bake until lightly browned, about 10 to 15 minutes. Remove the cookies from the baking sheet and let cool on wire racks.

Nutrition Facts Per Serving

- Cal 288
- GI 46
- Carb 35 g
- Fiber 3 g
- Protein 3 g
- Sodium 68 mg

Conclusion

With a healthy, balanced diet plan, you can lower or even eliminate menopause symptoms.